Advanced Jumping Using Water

High-Frequency Affinity to Attract Money, Love, Health and Attunement

Dr. Quantum

© Copyright 2021 - All rights reserved.

The content contained within this book may not be reproduced, duplicated or transmitted without direct written permission from the author or the publisher.

Under no circumstances will any blame or legal responsibility be held against the publisher, or author, for any damages, reparation, or monetary loss due to the information contained within this book, either directly or indirectly.

Legal Notice:

This book is copyright protected. It is only for personal use. You cannot amend, distribute, sell, use, quote or paraphrase any part, or the content within this book, without the consent of the author or publisher.

Disclaimer Notice:

Please note the information contained within this document is for educational and entertainment purposes only. All effort has been executed to present accurate, up to date, reliable, complete information. No warranties of any kind are declared or implied. Readers acknowledge that the author is not engaged in the rendering of legal, financial, medical or professional advice. The content within this book has been derived from various sources. Please consult a licensed professional before attempting any techniques outlined in this book.

By reading this document, the reader agrees that under no circumstances is the author responsible for any losses, direct or indirect, that are incurred as a result of the use of the information contained within this document, including, but not limited to, errors, omissions, or inaccuracies.

Table Of Content

Introduction 1
   Quantum Jumping And Quantum Physics 3
   What Has Water Got To Do With It? 6

Chapter 1: Dr. Masaru Emoto's Water Experiment .. 8
   Can Water Shapeshift? 10
   Water And The Power Of Thoughts 11
   What Exactly Happened In This Experiment? 14
   Summary 19

Chapter 2: Emoto's Work On The Miraculous Zamzam Water 20
   What Is Zamzam Water? 20
   What Sets Zamzam Water Apart? 23
   Drinking Water With An Intention 24
   Principles Of Prophet Muhammad For Drinking Water 25
   Summary 27

Chapter 3: Water Healing With Energy 29
   Instill Gratitude Into Water For Cooking 31

Therapeutic Bathing 31

Healing Showers 32

Immediate Healing Using A Cup Of Water 32

Overnight Grounded Intention Using Water 32

Use Glass 33

Summary 34

Chapter 4: Decoding Water 35

Water Has Memory 35

The Science Behind The Consciousness Of Water 37

Summary 41

Chapter 5: Seven Laws Govern The Universe 42

The Law Of Mentalism 42

The Law Of Correspondence 43

The Law Of Vibration 43

The Law Of Polarity 44

The Law Of Rhythm 46

The Law Of Cause And Effect 47

The Law Of Gender 48

Summary 49

Chapter 6: The Basics Of Jumping Dimensions 50

What Is Quantum Jumping? 51

Why Is Water An Integral Part Of This Method? . 53

Who Can Perform Quantum Jumping? 53

How Long Does It Take To Quantum Jump?.........54

Is It Harmful?..55

How Do I Know If I Want To Quantum Jump? 56

Summary 56

Chapter 7: Understanding A Quantum Jumping 58

How Does This Technique Work?.........................61

The Law Of Vibration - An In-Depth Look...........62

The Double-Slit Experiment And Quantum Jumping 64

Step 1: Solid Matter 64

Step 1: The Results 65

Step 2: Light Waves 65

Step 2: The Results 66

Step 3: Electrons 66

Step 3: The Results 67

Step 3: Hypotheses..67

Step 3: Under Observation 68

What Can Be Learned From These Experiments?.68

Why The Double-Slit Experiment Is So Important69

Quantum Entanglement 70

Water And Its Importance In This Method...........72

Summary 73

Chapter 8: How To Perform The Two-Glass Method For Quantum Jumping...74

Intentions You Should Hold While Performing The Two-Glass Method 74

When Should You Perform The Two-Glass Method? 76

The Two-Glass Method 77

The Method 77

Time And Place 81

Minimize Distractions 82

Before You Begin 83

Think About What You Want To Do 83

Start The Method 85

Think About What You Want To Change And Write It Down 85

Pour Water Into The Current State Glass 86

Current State 86

Forgiveness And Love 87

Place The Current State Cup Down 88

Desired State 88

Bless The Water 89

Place The Empty Cup Down And Thank The Divine Power 89

Summary 92

Chapter 9: The One-Glass Method 94

What Is The One-Glass Method? 96

What You'll Need 98

The One-Glass Method 99

Step 1: Your Desire(S) 99

Step 2: Set Your Intention 100

Step 3: Energize Yourself 101

Step 4: Visualize Your Future 102

Step 5: Return To The Present 102

Step 6: Go About Your Day 103

Am I Rich Yet? 103

Summary 105

Conclusion **106**

What To Take Away From These Experiences ... 109

References **111**

Introduction

When you hear the words "quantum jumping", what exactly comes to mind? If the words "quantum physics" spring to mind, you're on the right track. Do you think the word "quantum" immediately makes this book a possible science-fiction novel?

The answer to all of the above is that quantum jumping is indeed based on the concept of quantum physics, but it is not solely based on the studies of scientists in the quantum physics field. If you are interested in quantum jumping, then you need a better understanding of exactly what it entails and how to perform the jump that so many people have sworn works and are talking about.

First, you need to be introduced to the theory of the existence of multiverses, if you haven't been already.

This is the idea that we exist at the same time in multiple dimensions and universes but are leading either the same, worse, or better lives than in our current state or universe.

Quantum jumping is a technique that is used by many people around the world to visit their many different versions across all dimensions of the multiverse. It may sound like science-fiction, but there have been so many people who swear that they have met multiple versions of themselves as they performed quantum jumps to other universes in the multiverse.

People from completely different backgrounds, cultures, ages, and walks of life believe in the power of quantum jumping. With exciting new discoveries about water's ability to retain information, otherwise known as "water memory", the use of it to enhance the quantum jump experience is being noticed, and people are beginning to take advantage of it.

The fact that this technique is so simple and easy to perform is one of the many reasons why so many people are becoming interested in it. You will discover that the methods described are not only easy to perform but can be done by anyone. There are no harmful chemicals or substances needed—just you, the multiverse, some water, and all the energy that surrounds you.

Think of this book as an easy beginner's guide to

connecting to the version of yourself that will help you manifest the reality you have always wanted but never knew how to achieve.

Quantum Jumping and Quantum Physics

There are many thought processes when it comes to a viable definition of quantum physics. The Oxford dictionary describes it as the following: "The branch of physics concerned with quantum theory. Quantum physics allows for particles to be in two states at the same time" (Oxford, n.d.).

Stated simply, it's the physics study of how everything works and is the best means of describing all the millions of tiny particles that make up matter, as well as how they interact with one another. It describes how atomic particles work. Everything around us, including ourselves, is made up of these atomic particles—or in simple terms, matter. Quantum physics explains how biology and chemistry work.

Quantum physics is the study of how everything in our known universe works. Many famous scientists are renowned for their work as physicists. Some of these include the likes of:

- Isaac Newton
- Albert Einstein
- Niels Bohr
- Galileo Galilei

- Ernest Rutherford

There are many more names that can be added to this list of individuals who continue to do valuable research today to prove each of these great scientists and physicists who set the way forward for modern physicists today to continue with this work. One of these is Luc Montagnier, who was awarded the Nobel Prize for medicine after he discovered HIV. Today, he is much more interested in studying the effects of water when diluted DNA samples continue to be split to the point where no more DNA is present.

We will discuss this very interesting experiment in greater detail later; for now, just realize that water is currently receiving way more attention in all of the scientific spheres than ever before.

Modern physicists such as Stephen Hawking believed that multiple universes exist. This is what we will refer to as the multiverse. As I mentioned, quantum jumping takes qualities from the ideas and theories of quantum physics and incorporates spirituality and the human ability to manifest positive energy. It supports the idea of multiple universes and that there exist different versions of yourself in these alternate realities at the same time that you are existing in your current state. However, these other versions of you could either be at a better or worse stage in their life journey than you.

By tapping into their frequency, you can gain important knowledge from the different versions of you. You can then use whatever you have learned and apply it to your current state. Tapping into these various universes in the multiverse provides you with the extra energy that is needed for manifestation and also valuable information that can be applied to your current reality. The great thing is that the advice the multiverse version of you offers the current version of you comes from the experience of a trusted source: yourself.

People who have been even the most skeptical and cynical of quantum jumping using water have tried it, perhaps just because it sounded like it was something quite cool to do. Since then, it has become part of their daily routine. They have discovered exactly how powerful it can be.

As you begin to experience changes in your life—even small ones which you may not notice at first—it is a sign that you are shifting dimensions between where you are now and where you want to be. This is all achieved by channeling.

Channeling is the action of drawing energy from a power source. In this instance, it is the other version of you. This allows you to manifest what you ask for in this reality, because it exists in your parallel version's world. The positive energy that they are experiencing can be brought over to your current universe. You are connecting your energy in this universe to the energy of an infinite number of versions of you across dimensions. All of the energy that's channeled has great power.

As mentioned before, quantum jumping is something that can be done by anyone who is able to hold a clear intention of what they want. This book will introduce you to the basics of jumping using methods that have been around for centuries. Try and leave whatever skepticism you might have on this page, and as you read further, try and do so without prejudice as this will allow you to make a final decision about whether quantum jumping using water is for you.

What Has Water Got to Do With It?

Throughout the book, you will notice a distinct theme. I will speak about using water as part of your quantum jumping experience. Why water, though? Well, water has many healing properties. As one of the seven earthly elements, it holds a massive amount of energy on Earth. We see it as a sign of life—as the driving force of all existence. Therefore, it makes the perfect chemical structure for the energy you channel when you quantum jump.

Scientists have done studies that show how water can remember the molecular structure that was dissolved in it, even after that structure has been diluted with water. It was this very discovery that led to the use of water in quantum jumping, but we'll deal with all of this in more detail as we continue through the book.

Before you move on to Chapter 1, I want you to think about water—its flowing motion and the beautiful sounds it makes when it flows. Now imagine all of that flowing through you; feel the water inside your body flow. Imagine the feeling that you get when you drink a glass of cold water on a hot day. There is no better sensation than quenching your thirst.

If you managed to have those feelings and imagined the water on your lips traveling through you as a vivid image, then you're closer to understanding what it feels like to quantum jump.

Chapter 1
Dr. Masaru Emoto's Water Experiment

Let me start by asking you some simple yet conflicting questions:

- Do you believe that water has consciousness?
- Can water shapeshift?
- Can water react to thoughts?
- Can water remember?

I'm sure the immediate answer you came up with was no to these questions, and you might still be wondering how any of the above could take place. However, if you allow me to broaden your thinking, I can reveal to you the answers to the questions that seem impossible to comprehend.

Water is alive, and by alive, I mean it is conscious, and it exhibits consciousness by changing shapes, reacting to thoughts, and remembering what it came into contact with. Before going into specifics with regards to Dr. Masaru Emoto, we need to understand some of the scientific properties of water. Scientists, chemists, physicists, and various other subject matter experts will all agree that water possesses various chemical properties; these form polarity with one another (we'll consider the law of polarity a bit later, in Chapter 5). These molecules stick together like good friends at a party.

One of their other properties includes surface tension. In simplified terms, this means that because these water molecules all stick together, they can resist external forces or pressure. All of these facts have been proven by science through many studies and tests over hundreds of years.

What is a much newer theory, however, is that water is actually conscious and has the ability to remember things. There are several properties that water has that are not as clear-cut as each of the above theories. Part of these include water memory. Scientists and physicists are still trying to prove/disprove this theory, and the short answer is that in many instances, they aren't having all that much luck. The reason for this is that the moment water molecules realize they are being observed, they suddenly start behaving completely differently. How, then, are we supposed to prove scientifically that this is not just some random theory but that it's fact instead?

There's another piece of history here that is rather interesting, and it throws all of this research out on their heads. This is the fact that for years and years—centuries even—farmers and city planners had made use of what was commonly referred to as dowsing rods to find water sources underground. How these dowsing rods would work would be to react to two things: polarity and vibrational energy that the water molecules gave off. Sounds pretty cool, right?

Before we get to the actual experiments that made Dr. Emoto so famous, let's also take a quick look at some of the other questions above.

Can Water Shapeshift?

We know that water can shapeshift. All you have to do is pour water from one shaped receptacle to another shaped container, and it will immediately take exactly the same form as the container it's poured into. But that's not all; consider the way that a mountain stream or waterfall flows over boulders, rocks, and pebbles as it follows the natural course on its journey uphill or downhill.

Uphill? I hear you ask, "How can that be? Water cannot flow uphill." Believe it or not, a famous European logging merchant became fascinated by the way a river and waterway was able to propel heavy logs that should never have been able to float.

During his life, he created many designs to assist his logging business in moving logs from where they had been felled downstream to the actual lumber mill. His son and grandson have followed in his footsteps when it comes to the lumber business, but both have been fascinated by the movement of this water.

They have each concurred that water, in fact, spirals as it swirls over rocks and obstacles in its path. It creates furrows around obstacles added to the river bed. Due to erosion in the river and observing the natural path of the water, the grandson discovered that the water was densest and flowed fastest when it had obstacles such as rocks to move over and around.

He experimented by laying boulders all down the middle of the river bed to see what was going to happen. Working alongside geologists and water specialists at the local university, they were able to plot exactly what was happening to the riverbed. Sure enough, the water moved to the middle of the river, preferring to flow over the rocks and boulders that were added. This, in turn, created a natural habitat for the trout in the region.

Water and the Power of Thoughts

Water is able to react to thoughts. All you need to do is verify and study some of the experiments by Dr.

Masaru Emoto we have outlined below. Each one proves that both thought and intention can have an extremely powerful effect on the best quality water. The water that had been blessed or prayed over provided some of the most exquisite images of change to the molecular structure of water throughout these studies.

It all started with an experiment conducted by the renowned Japanese scientist, Dr. Masaru Emoto. He began his experiment at a time when he made use of water with the intent to cure people's diseases. The experiment began when Dr. Emoto observed the crystal structure of water to gain physical evidence that would prove water reacted to its surroundings and, therefore, could be used for more than healing.

While conducting his experiment, he came across a book about the crystal structure of a snowflake. That was the beginning of his curiosity and the driving force that led him to uncover the true nature of water that is hidden from the world. It gave him the idea to freeze the water and then use it to view the crystal structure of it under a very powerful microscope. Thus, water crystal technology came into being.

In 1990, Dr. Emoto was first introduced to working with water, filling different jars and containers and simply sticking various notes on each one. Some of these notes were positive, stating things like "Thank you", "I love you", "I care about you", and a whole slew of other uplifting thoughts. However, on others, the notes would be negative, stating things such as "I hate you", "You disgust me", or "I want to kill you".

After these bottles of water had been standing a while, he would take a single drop of water from each one, place these on individual slides, and freeze them until they formed crystals.

Apart from writing letters or words on pieces of paper, he would also play music to the water. Some of these tunes ranged from Mozart to heavy metal. Once again, the results were almost identical to the experiment above.

Not everyone has been a fan of his work and have argued that "given the high water composition of the human brain and body, if water is, in fact, conscious and receptive to energy frequencies, how can these positive or negative messages affect our bodies on a molecular level?"

What was displayed by each crystal under the microscope could hardly be explained. All the water that had positive intentions directed its way in the form of either calming and peaceful words or music that was refined displayed beautiful asymmetrical crystal formations.

Conversely, water droplets that had been frozen from jars containing words that were unkind or had experienced heavy metal music resulted in crystals that were no longer asymmetrical. As a matter of fact, most of these crystals were deformed and distorted. They looked nowhere near as interesting and unique as the other crystals (Mitte Team, 2019).

What Exactly Happened in This Experiment?

Dr. Masaru Emoto collected several water samples from various places and exposed them to different forms of positive and negative energy. These water droplets were then frozen so their crystal structures could be evaluated under a microscope. What's so intriguing about this experiment is that each of the water structures was different.

For instance, water collected from a river source that was polluted showed a distorted, asymmetrical, and unappealing structure. On the other hand, water collected from a clean stream and introduced to positive emotions and energy showed up in an almost symmetrical form as a beautiful composition with a ring in the middle and bright colors.

He didn't stop there, however. He then collected two samples from the Fujiwara dam: one before the Buddhists began to pray and one after. Surprisingly, the sample taken before the prayer showed no clear, symmetrical structure, but the sample which was taken after the prayer showed a clean, symmetrical, and beautiful geometric structure. The source from which the water was obtained remained the same, but the timing when it was extracted from the source was changed. It was incredible that a single hour-long prayer could transform the crystal structure to such an extent.

Dr. Emoto then took samples of water that were exposed to different thoughts—once again, both positive and negative. The results were unbelievable and showed a similar pattern to that of the Fujiwara Dam experiment. The water samples that were exposed to negative phrases showed deformed, wholly dissolved, and uneven crystal formation. However, the water samples that were exposed to positive words resulted in the most beautiful crystal structures.

This showed Dr. Emoto that positive words produced vibrant, well-defined, symmetrical, and pleasing physical structures, while negative energy or words caused the crystal structures to display asymmetrical structures that were unappealing to the eye.

Similar results were found when water was exposed to music. Peaceful symphonies of Mozart and other classical music produced hexagonal, symmetrical structures, but heavy metal music resulted in deformed, distorted, and minor crystal formations. It was not just music, though; water reacted the same way to images being shown to it. An image of a negative word shown to the water led to an unpleasant-looking structure, and a positive, happy image created a beautiful, appealing crystal structure.

It was clear from this experiment that water could perceive feelings and emotions communicated in any form, whether it was via words, thoughts, pictures, music, vibrations, or even touch.

To everyone's surprise, another experiment displayed that water holds memory. When a flower was dropped in a container of water and its samples were frozen, the crystal structure of the water sample replicated the flower. It is an unbelievable yet remarkable fact that water has a living consciousness.

The ability of water to hold memory is fascinating. In one case, a drop of flower oil was added to the water, and the crystal structure displayed the structure of the flower the oil came from. It is quite mind-boggling to even think about, but it shows the extent to which water can perceive and react.

This experiment opened new horizons in the field of quantum physics. It led us to really see how perceptive and sensitive matter can be. We cannot be oblivious to the fact that it can detect our intentions, even with the slightest hint. Water forms about 60% of our body mass and 71% of the earth's surface. It would be foolish of us to believe that our intentions, thoughts, words, and actions don't impact our life, health, and well-being

(USGS Science for a changing world, 2019).

Dr. Emoto began his water research while studying at the Open International University where he earned a doctorate in alternative medicine in 1992. It was there that he was introduced to micro-clusters of water. This began his subsequent obsession with the miracles that could be discovered in water. It was also at that time when he invented the water healing practice that is commonly referred to as Hado today. The very name Hado in Japanese translates to "move" or "wave". Dr. Emoto referred to Hado as "the intrinsic vibrational pattern at the atomic level in all matter. The smallest unit of energy. Its basis is the energy of human consciousness" (The Spirit of Life, n.d.).

Hado as described by Dr. Emoto on the official Hado website explains how everything gives off energy, an aura, even thoughts and feelings. These things interact and influence everything else around them. Remember speaking about the universe not being in a vacuum, but rather being filled with matter. Matter is all around us vibrating at different frequencies.

Depending on the level of these vibrations, frequencies can be influenced to change these things. Stimuli could come from anything, including thought, speech, and music. Each of these vibrations would have an effect on the matter, especially water since it holds memory. In the tests that Dr. Emoto conducted with water, he compared human emotions (how we would feel) with the way that water reacted to the same situation.

Consider how you feel when someone is kind to you and they smile. You feel good about yourself, right? Now, how do you feel when someone is rude or insults you? You feel the opposite to the above. Let's face it, none of us enjoy being called out or made to feel small and unimportant.

His tests included the written word as well, and this is where it becomes fascinating because water can respond to written matter. Is this all sounding a bit bizarre and far-fetched for you right now? Keep reading with an open mind.

Many of the above experiments involved freezing water with words taped to the container that read things like "I love you", "thank you", or "I hate you". As each of these containers froze and were examined under his microscope, he describes the positive words as creating the most beautiful crystal shapes while negative concepts produced structures that looked as though they were totally deformed.

Hado was used as a form of Japanese healing utilizing water. Dr. Emoto found this through his studies with water and proceeded with using water infused with positive emotions for healing. He would consult with individuals who were experiencing negative problems in their lives, offering them an alternative method of healing through his water technique. His work was acclaimed for years, and the practice of Hado is still attributed to his work. It has been associated with homeopathy.

Hado teaches that positive thinking is a practice where health, vitality, and positive thinking are beneficial to the recipient of this water.

Summary

By analyzing the crystal structure of water, we are able to see the quantum level changes in it. These transformations are due to vibrations, emotions, images, spoken and written words, thoughts, and actions.

We are still unable to trace how or why water reacts to our thoughts, but studying the changes in the crystal structures of water is the closest we have ever come to evaluating matter at this level. If water is so receptive to everything around it, imagine how sensitive matter itself can be.

Chapter 2:
Emoto's Work on the Miraculous Zamzam Water

In the previous chapter, we discovered that water has consciousness. It is capable of understanding and memorizing thoughts, emotions, words, pictures, vibrations, and music. In this chapter, we will move on to Zamzam water and its unique properties. We briefly spoke about the healing techniques of Hado, where curing takes place through water. We also discussed renowned researcher, Dr. Emoto.

This chapter will explore and help you understand how Zamzam water helps with healing and the power involved in assigning an intention to water.

What Is Zamzam Water?

We saw how the crystal structure of water from the Fujiwara Dam was transformed after being exposed to prayers. Does this mean that the holy water from a different source will show the same result? The following experiment conducted by Dr. Emoto answers this question.

The holy water of followers of the Prophet Mohammad is known as Zamzam water. It has an intriguing and miraculous history as well as other properties such as its origin, the speed at which it flows, its pH, and its crystalline structure. We will focus more on each of these distinct properties later. To begin with, let me give you some deeper insight into Zamzam water.

The Well of Zamzam is in the Masjid al-Haram in Mecca, Saudi Arabia, 20 meters east of the Kaaba, which is the holiest place in Islam ("Zamzam Studies and Research Centre" Saudi Geological Survey (in Arabic)). The word is derived from "zome zome", meaning "stop flowing".

Zamzam water first originated thousands of years ago when Ishmael, the son of Hagar and Abraham, was crying of thirst in the desert. It is believed that the spring of water appeared as a token of love for Ishmael from God.

The spring of water is known as the initial source of Zamzam water. Historical documents place this wellspring discovery at around 1910 BCE. Casting your mind back, or using a calculator, you will note that this water has been flowing underground for more than 4,000 years. It's believed that the source of water in the Zamzam well is due to the well being a renewable source. Mecca receives a lot of rain, and it is in one of these valleys that the Zamzam Well is located in a low-lying area, according to Sharaqi (Akkawi, 2018).

Geologically, it has taken millions of years for this well to be created. This water is sacred to anyone completing their annual pilgrimage to Mecca. It is only for drinking for those visiting Mecca, especially for Hajj and Umrah pilgrims. During these pilgrimages, millions of liters of this special water are consumed (Staff Writer Al Arabiya, 2018).

The water has been flowing non-stop for thousands of years and has never dried up. It consistently maintains the same levels of salts and minerals to date. It is considered to be a pure and unadulterated source of water, and it has many healing properties due to its high salt content (sodium, magnesium) and an alkaline pH.

Part of the reason why Zamzam water will never dry up, according to geology professor Abbas Sharaqi, is because it is connected to a renewable source of groundwater. The only time this water could be potentially threatened would be under extreme geological conditions (Akkawi, 2018).

Zamzam water has a pH range of 7.2 to 8.0, which is highly alkaline and the best water for human consumption. Apart from its pH and salt content, the crystal structure of the Zamzam water is one of a kind.

What Sets Zamzam Water Apart?

Dr. Masaru Emoto was looking for a type of water that was pure and couldn't be tainted by magic. How could a scientist possibly believe in magic and spells? Well, when you witness water behaving like a conscious person, you end up analyzing all the possibilities. He wanted to check if the influence of magic or spells was the cause of the distinct behavior witnessed during his research. Therefore, he decided to test water that is known to be immune to magic, spells, and external influences. That's when one of his colleagues recommended Zamzam water, stating that it could not be influenced by magic or spells.

Dr. Emoto started trying to freeze the Zamzam water but failed. It was unable to solidify and form a crystal structure, so he started to dilute it. Finally, when he diluted the water to one drop to a 1,000-ml ratio, the crystal structure was finally achieved.

The structure it formed was unlike anything else he had ever seen before. Through his experiment, he found that it formed an overlapping twin structure. He also tried to play the verses of the Holy Quran to the water, and the crystal structure replicated the shape of Mecca. He went on to discover that each name of Allah produced a different yet beautiful structure. Dr. Emoto was sure that Zamzam water had unique properties and was pure.

After the completion of Dr. Emoto's research, he started practicing Hado. He healed people by having them drink water that he had added positive intentions to. After his research, he learned a lot about the fascinating healing properties of water. This made it easier for him to understand the mechanism of action of water in the human body, and this was reflected in his healing methods.

His research was so successful that to this day, he will always be remembered for his practice of Hado. Let's take a more in-depth look at how associating intentions can lead to healing.

Drinking Water With an Intention

Water these days travels over thousands of miles to reach our homes, and almost all sources of this necessity are polluted in some way. The water in our glass is devoid of active energy. Pollution, toxicity, stagnating in dark pipes, and treating it with chemicals strips the water of all its nourishing and active energy. Even the crystal structure of water changes. So, we aren't drinking water in its purest state at all.

Even when an animal is given the choice to drink

water from a natural spring or a tap, the animal will always choose to drink from a spring. Naturally, it seems fresher and higher in energy to the animal. Zamzam water holds this pure state because it is constantly flowing. It also happens to be close to a religious place brimming with prayers and positive energy. This is what causes Zamzam water to be so pure.

Water in its normal state is neutral. It does, however, take on the properties of whatever it comes into contact with. Whenever we drink water without any intention, it flows through our body, coming into contact with everything in our current state. This could be illnesses, negativity, sadness, or despair. This water becomes part of that and begins to vibrate at the same level as each of these negative emotions. It becomes one with whatever we are holding on to.

Some other negative emotions might include, anger, grief, and physical pain. It is only when we assign positive intentions with water that we can help ourselves overcome the negative effects of disease and illness. While this may have been something new to Dr. Emoto, the followers of Muhammad have been practicing these methods for thousands of years.

Principles of Prophet Muhammad for Drinking Water

The Prophet Muhammad asks his followers to

remember God, or Allah, before drinking the Zamzam water and to express gratitude after drinking the water. The first step is what associates an intention with the water. Drinking it in the name of God or Allah is to drink to the creator of the universe or for the one ultimate source of energy. This curbs any negative effects the water may be carrying, and by aligning your intention with the water, it no longer mixes with all the diseases and negativities your body may be holding on to, instead healing the mind, body, and soul.

The second step is to be conscious of the water and recognize that it is thanks to God, Allah, or the universe that we have the gift of water to drink. The gift of water is the gift of life. Without water, we would not be able to survive. Take time to contemplate this.

Thanking God or Allah after drinking the water connects us to the divine intention of love via gratitude. When we offer our thanks for the water, we enter a state of thankfulness wherein we surrender to the intent we associated with the water and allow the changes to take place.

Associating visualization and emotional intention while keeping in the mind the creator of the universe will enhance the quality of the water. Water travels miles and miles to reach us. The energy is low; the chemical structure is altered. When we pray over it and bless it while remembering the creator, its structure changes, and it activates the energy in water. That is why associating intent with water is essential. Doing so can heal us, lift our moods, and nourish us.

Our bodies are 60% water, and there must be a reason for that. Even water flows in, throughout, and out of our bodies. It can surely cleanse, rejuvenate, heal, and uplift the aura of a person. Thus, we mustn't neglect water or keep drinking it without intention. Our thoughts and prayers have the ability to re-energize and restructure water into its pure state.

The Prophet Muhammad recommends drinking water in slow sips rather than gulping it down as you might do when you are very thirsty on a hot day. The intention should be to take note of the water as it enters and flows throughout your body. It is suggested that at least three breaths be taken in between sipping the water from your glass.

There are several other instructions that the Prophet Muhammad instructed Muslims and non-Muslims to follow. These are simply to be seated when you drink water rather than standing as well as starting and ending the entire process with a prayer.

Summary

Dr. Emoto proved with his research that one drop of Zamzam water can turn 1,000 ml of ordinary water into Zamzam water. It is a sign of the purity of water. Even if the quality of water we drink is outstanding, how we drink it is even more crucial. We learned that like the followers of Prophet Mohammad, even Dr. Emoto associated counteracting intentions to the water for healing purposes. Our emotions, thoughts, ideas, prayers, and intent can give water the ability to heal us at the quantum level. Hold on to the word quantum, as we are going to discuss why it is so important and what its relation to water and our overall well-being is.

Chapter 3: Water Healing With Energy

We've already discussed that water is necessary for any living thing on this planet to survive. Without it, the world as we know it would cease to exist. Did you know that it has been revered by individuals throughout history? "Water healing ceremonies" have been conducted to heal plants, people, and animals throughout the annals of time. The main reason for this is due to its therapeutic properties. Water retains whatever it is exposed to. Whether good or bad, positive or negative intentions, toxic chemicals, or the purest form possible, water retains whatever it comes into contact with.

Dr. Emoto made the following statement in his New York Bestselling Book, *The Hidden Messages in Water*: "If we have a clear understanding of water, we will better understand the human body and even unlock the mystery of why we were born" (Emoto, 2004).

Water surrounds us constantly. It's in the air we breathe. It falls to Earth in the form of rain and snow. It takes up a majority of the earth in terms of oceans, lakes, rivers, and streams. It can often be found in the form of fresh, natural springs. Because everything that's living needs water to survive and thrive, you will even find water in the food we eat.

Imagine being able to harness the healing energy of all this water daily? Well, you can, as long as you set your intention and truly believe. You can charge anything that contains water with vibrational energy from the universe and even the multiverse. You can physically charge anything containing water with gratitude, prayers, healing, light energy, or any intention you choose to set.

Long before the groundbreaking discoveries of Dr. Emoto, Amazonian tribes would sing as a way to charge water with energy necessary for healing. Other tribes and nations around the world have been participating in rain dances. Water is also central to many religious ceremonies and sacred rites such as baptisms, cleansings, healing, and even the act of blessing and sanctifying water to make it holy.

According to traditional Reiki healer Corie Chu, there are a number of very basic healing ceremonies that can be done using water. Each of these is easy to do, and you don't need fancy equipment or paraphernalia.

Instill Gratitude Into Water for Cooking

We use water for doing anything from cooking rice, boiling potatoes, steaming vegetables, and making various other culinary dishes. Before beginning any food preparation using water, we should express gratitude. This is done through a prayer over water you will use to cook anything you would eat yourself or over food you are cooking for others. Your prayer can include a request that it heals the bodies of those that eat anything cooked using this water.

Therapeutic Bathing

A normal bathing experience can be turned into something both therapeutic and healing. Instead of just routinely bathing, fill the bathtub with warm water, adding your choice of essential oils, flowers, or milk. You can further enhance this experience by lighting candles or incense. Add music to this experience (suitable for meditation). Instead of playing music in the background, you may want to bless the water with a prayer.

Submerge yourself in the water slowly, settle back by closing your eyes, and take time to meditate. Don't rush your bathing ritual. Take the time to cleanse every part of your body.

Healing Showers

Have you ever felt as though the weight of the world is on your shoulders? Have you felt the anxiety of someone you've recently been speaking with? Regardless of whether you are dirty or not, you can use a shower as a means of washing all forms of negativity away. If you know that you absorb energy from others, this would be especially beneficial for you. Doing so at the end of the day will help you sleep better.

Immediate Healing Using a Cup of Water

Pour a glass of water. While holding it between your hands, channel your intention with what you would like to bless. Visualize your intention being transferred to the water. This is a vital step. You should be able to imagine every cell of the water being filled with your healing intention.

When you are certain that your intention is firmly fixed, breathe deeply and take your first drink of the water. As you sit, imagine the intention that you've set into the water being transported throughout your body. Once you have completed this process, take the next sip of water and repeat the same visualization technique as outlined above. Repeat this until the water is finished or for as long as you like.

Overnight Grounded Intention Using Water

This is similar to the initial process with the

exception that you bless the water before leaving it overnight for anywhere between 10 and 12 hours. Visualize healing light throughout the water before drinking any of it. There are several variations to this intention. You can write out a prayer and physically tie it around the bottle or container that the water is in. You would still leave this overnight.

Before retiring for the evening, read through the prayer and intention and wrap it around the bottle once more. It's important that the bottle you use is made of glass.

Use Glass

Plastic bottles contain all sorts of chemicals such as bisphenol, more commonly known as (BPA), that can contaminate the water. BPA is toxic, and due to food processing and plastic containers we use almost daily, each of us has various levels of BPA detectable in our systems.

In the morning, repeat the prayer, affirmation, or intention before drinking any of this water. As you do so, concentrate on feeling the vibrational energy moving through every inch of your body. Imagine this healing energy being able to cleanse and heal every cell within you at an atomic level (Chu, 2020; National Capital Poison Centre, n.d.).

Another much more practical reason for using glass

rather than plastic is that it is actually made from an earth element, sand. While it is not in its natural state, it makes logical sense that earth and water are going to work much better together than water in a potentially contaminated plastic container. Anything that represents one of the natural elements can be used; this would include wood and metal (also known as ether).

Summary

In this chapter, we have discovered that there are various simple healing methods we can easily perform on our own in our homes or wherever necessary. We discovered that as we bless or speak to the water, vibrational changes take place, and water has the ability to take on distinctive healing properties simply through thought and intention.

We have also learned that it is better to make use of glass instead of plastics because water can take on the properties of whatever it is placed in. BPA is poisonous, and glass is made from sand, yet another element that is connected to the universe.

Chapter 4: Decoding Water

So far, you have read that water has consciousness. It can reciprocate emotions by changing its molecular structure, and it has memory. Dr. Emoto proved the theory by taking pictures of the variations in the molecular structure of the water once frozen or close to being frozen, but the reason why this happens is still unclear. So, here is some scientific proof and observation for you.

Water Has Memory

Water can hold memory. It can copy the image of an object, feelings, and thoughts it comes in contact with, but is there more to it? We have only read a small page of a huge and heavy book. There is a lot to understand, interpret, and ponder upon. There is more to water that remains untouched and undiscovered. You would be surprised to know that water can copy electromagnetic signals, vibrations, pathogenic DNA, and whatever it comes into contact with. Yes, that is a shocking admission but entirely true. If water can hold on to emotions, it can hold on to frequencies and electromagnetic inputs, too. It can effortlessly copy the radio signals emitted by the pathogenic DNA.

A Nobel Prize-winning virologist, Luc Montagnier, has experimented with water using the DNA of bacterial and viral pathogens. The remarkable fact is that after diluting the pathogens to the point where they were hardly even detectable, the water was able to produce similar electromagnetic signals to the DNA.

I know you must be thinking that DNA came in contact with water and water copied it. Well, that is the right assumption based on what you've learned so far, but there is more data to back it. Get ready to be more surprised than you already are.

The electromagnetic signals were converted into audio waves or radio waves and sent from the lab in Germany where Luc Montagnier was all the way to another top virology lab in France. Here, it was carefully ensured that the water that was going to be tested for the memory didn't come in contact with the DNA at all. Receiving the soundwaves via email, the lab in France played the audio file for an hour to a brand-new vial of sterile water that had not been touched nor tampered with. You need to pay great attention at this point, because the water the audio was played to had only ever been in contact with the audio or the radio waves.

When this sample of water was tested, it gave the same electromagnetic signals, and almost identical DNA radio signals were achieved. Tests conducted at a third independent laboratory confirmed that the sample received via the audio file from Germany was a 98% match to the DNA audio file in France. If this doesn't prove the power of water to you, I'm not sure what will. It is fascinating how water can display such consciousness.

The Science Behind the Consciousness of Water

Water has a chemical structure of H2O. It has two molecules of hydrogen and one molecule of oxygen. Even a drop of water contains thousands of H2O molecules. When H2O molecules become tightly packed together, the oxygen molecules are able to link together, forming a tight circular structure. Once in this circular structure, they prevent anything from passing through. This is how water is able to retain memory, displaying a level of consciousness that still continues to baffle scientists today.

They are so tightly packed that the H2O structure forms a circular structure. It thus forms a void in the middle of the structure. Of course, the voids in the water droplet are made at a quantum level. It is these voids, aka empty spaces in water, that copy, memorize, and bear consciousness. At the quantum level even, water is made with the same energy and same quantum particles as the universe. It is these quantum particles that are responsible for the nature of water.

Water is the only compound found in nature that has a molecular structure which expands when it freezes. Under normal conditions, molecules will contract when they get cold. What's more, according to a professor in physics and director of the Physics Institute at Brazil's Universidade Federal do Rio Grande do Sul, Marcia Barbosa, they behave completely differently from any other substance on Earth.

She explains how during winter, rivers and lakes freeze over with a dense layer of ice, while under the ice is a pocket of water that's approximately zero degrees. This pocket of water is still very cold but below it, it has a third layer of water that's just above the riverbed. Here, the water temperature is warm and sustains whatever fish and aquatic life forms need to survive. How awesome is it that water knows exactly how much space is needed to support life underwater? (TEDxCERN & Barbosa, 2014).

Water is programmable, and that is why all forms of life include water. Water is the sole thing we look for when we search for life on other planets. It is capable of preserving vibration, imitating the same character as it is shown or communicated to.

A scientist who is working on water memory believes that if their experiments continue to progress, then water could be used as an alternative to medicine. Imagine if water could copy pathogenic DNA and emit the same radio signals; it could also copy the chemical structure of medicines and produce the same results as them. After all, if the water molecules can preserve the structure of medicine, they could produce similar effects in the body.

Programming water at such a level will be cost-effective, easy to use, and less toxic for everyone. It may take years to program water at such a level for mass use, but we can do it at home for our benefit.

If we talk about the composition of the human body, you would be surprised to know that 75% of our brains are made of water. Why is it made up of water? This is solely because water can sense vibrations, feelings, thoughts, and intentions; it has an abundance of omniscient energy and can quickly transition into any desired state.

We are conscious beings that think, feel, perceive, and dream, and that is why the brain is made up of mostly water. Our mind is receptive and continuously interacts with the universe at a quantum level.

If our bodies consist of such high percentages of

water and we are able to control what happens to the water before we consume it, then surely we have the power to transform some of the water within our own systems. Think about the experiment where the single DNA strand was diluted, and diluted, and diluted ten times over until there was no trace of DNA. What if we were able to raise the vibrational energy throughout our bodies from 60% to 75%? How much of a difference would we be able to make within our own lives?

We can do this simply by following the methods below on quantum water jumping. It is indeed possible to heal yourself through the intentions that you put out into the multiverses.

The brain is an expert at utilizing the water that flows through it. Not just to understand emotions and save memories, this water is also used to cure certain disorders. When one part of the brain fails to function effectively due to a minor injury or accident, water transports the action to another part of the organ that acts as a substitute. It memorizes the function and feeds it to another part of the brain, and the action continues without interruption. Even our conscious and subconscious memories are based on water.

The memories that stay grounded in the subconscious part of the brain are there because the water carries them there. You only experience and feel these memories when the subconscious state is activated during yoga or meditation, or while listening to serene music that allows your body to relax into a trance-like state.

Summary

I hope this proof was able to establish more confidence in you about the powers of water. The ability of it to heal at a quantum level is unmatched. All you need to do is to program it with the right intention. In the next few chapters, we will learn how water can be a medium for us to achieve total well-being in all areas of life.

Chapter 5:
Seven Laws Govern the Universe

The universe has seven laws that govern it and everything around it. Everything in the universe consists of vibrations, frequencies, and energies. These seven laws are covered in this chapter.

The first three of these laws are immutable. This means that they are fixed, eternal, and cannot be altered in any way.

The Law of Mentalism

All things that exist throughout the multiverse were created by a higher power through the divine mind of the Source. Whether you refer to this divine mind as God, Allah, or any other higher being that you revere, understand that it is eternal and will always be eternal. Everything was created through this great will.

You can harness all of this energy and power into your own life by focusing your attention and thoughts on those things that you want to attract. Some of these things might include peace, love, abundance, friendship, joy, or career success. Whatever you choose to focus your intention on will become a reality in your present life.

The Law of Correspondence

The second immutable law is the Law of correspondence. This one is based on the theory of "as above, so below; as below, so above". It confirms a connection between heaven and Earth, the spiritual and mental realms. Whatever is happening on the outside must correspond with what's happening on the inside. When we are facing inner conflict, we will always see the same thing manifest in our lives externally.

To gain the most from working with this law, you need to take care of what's happening within you. Until your life is filled with peace and joy internally, you cannot expect the rest of your world to become the way you truly want it to be. Deal with your inner emotions and turmoil first, and the rest will fall into place.

The Law of Vibration

The final immutable law is the law of vibration. It states that everything throughout the universe and multiverse vibrates at a frequency. Everything consists of energy. Depending on what's happening in your life, this energy can either be at a high-frequency vibration or low-frequency vibration.

This is the law that people refer to when they speak of the law of attraction. This clearly states that whatever you focus on and put out there with intention is exactly what will come back to you. This refers not only to your words and deeds, but to your thoughts and emotions as well.

The famous physicist Albert Einstein said, "Everything is energy. Match the frequency of the reality you want, and you cannot help but get that reality. There can be no other way. This is not philosophy. This is physics."

The law of attraction simply cannot deny you what you put out into the multiverse with intention. Understand that the laws of the universe are always working *for* us, not against us.

The following four laws are all mutable, which basically means that they are forever changing. They are never in a constant state and can shift whenever necessary.

The Law of Polarity

The first of the four mutable laws is the one of polarity. The mutable laws are never in a constant state and can shift whenever necessary.

Everything has a polar opposite. For there to be day, there needs to be night; for happiness, sadness, for joy, there needs to be pain. The Kybalion explains it like this: "Everything is dual; everything has poles; everything has its pairs of opposites; like and unlike are the same; opposites are identical in nature, but different in degree; extremes meet; all truths are but half-truths; all paradoxes may be reconciled."

Through duality, we can see that the above things are the same, just at different degrees of one another. Where we currently see opposites, these are really just another version of the same. Think of positive and negative, love and fear, light and dark.

We need to understand that this law only exists in the mental and physical realms. Everything is one in the spiritual realm. For your life to be perfectly balanced, you need to find balance between the two. This is done by consciously raising your vibrational state. We've briefly spoken about vibrations, but I'm going to go into greater detail about how to use them to your advantage.

The middle path within the law of polarity is the path of peace. This is where every intention and thought that you have and every word that you utter should be focused on the divine creator of the universe, whether you refer to this being as God, Allah, or anything else you want to call it. Some people directly refer to the universe as such itself.

The Law of Rhythm

The next law is one of rhythm. The pendulum of our lives continues to swing back and forth constantly. Everything has a natural order and rhythm attached. Once again, these wise words come from the Kybalion: "Everything flows, out and in; everything has its tides; all things rise and fall; the pendulum-swing manifests in everything; the measure of the swing to the right is the measure of the swing to the left; rhythm compensates."

Consider your chest rising and falling as you breathe in oxygen and breathe out carbon dioxide. There are cycles within nature; spring becomes summer, summer becomes autumn, autumn turns into winter, and the cycle begins again. There are phases to the moon and different phases to the tides. Relationships begin and end, and there's a time to be born and a time to die. These rhythms are constantly happening throughout the multiverse.

We sometimes become confused and fearful when the pendulum happens to be swinging in the wrong direction for us. Instead of hitting the panic button, this is where we should become excited in knowing that we are right on the cusp of things turning for us. The pendulum cannot suddenly stop; it must follow the natural order of things. So, too, our lives must be filled with both good times and bad, and the cycle commences once again.

The Law of Cause and Effect

Cause and effect is a law of accountability and consequence. For every action, there needs to be a similar reaction. Every cause has an effect, and every effect has a cause. The secret is discovering that every thought we put out there will be returned to us. We can sometimes be very disappointed with the effect of this law. Some of the consequences to our thoughts and actions are hard to swallow. The power lies in what we choose to think about and the strength of our intention.

Although cause and effect exist on all three planes of existence, on the spiritual plane they happen instantly. There's a time delay on the physical and mental planes. All that this means is that we have no idea when the consequences of our decisions and actions will occur. Some happen immediately, while others take place many years down the line.

Working with this law means that you should understand that everything you think, say, and do will have an impact on you at some point. Your thoughts materialize as your reality, and what you choose to focus on becomes your reality.

You need to set your goals clearly with intention

while ignoring all the other negative thoughts trying to take over your mind. With clear, focused intention, consider each of your goals, dismissing every negative thought the moment one appears. This means being able to physically visualize your goals and your desired intention so that the universe is able to work with you to manifest exactly what you want.

You may question whether you have the ability to change your reality from where you are now. All you really need to do is to focus your intention with nothing wavering, and your greatest desires will begin to show up.

The Law of Gender

The final law of the universe is the law of gender. Creation could not exist without this law. It can be found across every living species and even down to molecular structures and the charging of energy fields. Psychologically, we have both male and female qualities. However, physically, we are connected to our material form in the gender in which we were created.

There are yin and yang in each of us; we each possess heavenly aspects of both sets of qualities. When you consider female qualities, you probably think about things such as love, compassion, kindness, patience, and understanding. Males, on the other hand, are best known for their ability to use their intellect and logic. Finding the delicate balance between these two can lead us on our path to success and enlightenment (Ismail, 2020).

Summary

There are seven major laws that are laws of the universe. Some of them are immutable, meaning that they are permanent; they cannot be changed. The final four laws can be changed and operate according to things happening around us all the time. We are not surrounded by nothingness. Instead, we have atomic particles, energy, and matter all around us. Everything is constantly vibrating, which is exactly how water can be energized through these vibrations.

The most important law, which is actually a combination of all seven of these laws, is the law of attraction. Once we understand this, we are able to set our intention to the universe much quicker.

Chapter 6: The Basics of Jumping Dimensions

We live in a universe of infinite possibilities, and it is rightly said that you could achieve whatever you want for yourself or others. In the past few chapters, you have read about how water at a molecular level is alive, programmable, and capable of retaining memory. Let us now talk about water at the quantum level.

When we talk about quantum, we are essentially talking about things at a cellular and subatomic level. For an atom, the quantum level is an electron, and for us, it would be a single cell of our body. Why are we talking in quantum terms? Well, because it is only at the quantum level that we can find the answers to why things are a certain way in this universe.

If we look at things at a quantum level, only then can we understand the miracles of the universe. Quantum is the core of the universe. It is one of the most sought-after yet least explored areas in the field of science. It also happens to be one area of science and physics where there are still many answers to be found. The building blocks of the universe, and even ourselves, all sit in the quantum realm.

What Is Quantum Jumping?

Quantum jumping is a method that can help you jump dimensions and achieve almost anything that your heart desires. If what I just said sounds like science-fiction, then allow me to break it down for you as something backed with the ideas of the studies of the universe.

We live in multiverses and not in a universe. There exists an outcome for every single thing that you do or aspire to do. I guess that's where we got the sayings, "You reap what you sow", and, "What goes around comes around". Despite doing your best, you don't get results and think the best is not happening for you. But what if it is?

In the multiverses, energy is conserved and simply transferred from one dimension to another. This means that the efforts that you put in one dimension are reflecting in another. Why does that sound similar to Newton's Law? It's because that's exactly what it is! If you are not at your best in one dimension, you might be an emperor in another. Sounds unbelievable, right? Continue reading, and I guarantee that you will start believing, too.

Currently, in this universe, let's suppose you earn a minimal salary and you happen to be a sickly person. But in another universe and another dimension, you are a rich person who has a perfectly healthy body. You can be a painter, writer, dancer, athlete, billionaire, or any other version of yourself that you can possibly imagine. There exists '**n**' numerous universes and there exists '**n**' numerous variations of you. These multiverses exist simultaneously in real-time along with you. It is only through our consciousness that we can tap into these dimensions and choose to be any version of ourselves. That is the essence of quantum jumping.

Quantum jumping is a leap of our consciousness from our current state to the desired state using visualization as the medium. You can choose to acquire a new trait, enhance your current lifestyle, gain health, or enrich your life in any conceivable way possible, and you can do it all by quantum jumping. This is not magic or a vague idea that has no base. This is a scientifically-backed theory and works perfectly. Before we learn the method of quantum jumping, let's learn a bit about some laws of the universe and things to keep in mind. Once you understand quantum jumping at a quantum level, it will be easier for you to jump dimensions.

Why Is Water an Integral Part of This Method?

Water is alive and gives life. It has the ability to understand and capture our real emotions genuinely. It can help us take the quantum leap, as it has the capability to transition at a quantum level. It can harness and transition emotions, feelings, and thoughts at a cellular level and because of this it can help us take the quantum leap from our current state to the desired state. It also does this job effectively, easily, and quickly. There is no scope of mishap or failure. It's the safest medium that you can use for the job.

Who Can Perform Quantum Jumping?

Anyone is able to jump dimensions using the following methods of quantum jumping I will be sharing with you. You don't have to be a saint, an ardent believer of God, or a religious preacher to do it, nor do you have to levitate in the air or sacrifice anything to achieve the results you want out of life. It is very simple to do if you understand the main concept and accept it.

All you need is a clear understanding of the method and a strong consciousness to perform the task. This strong will is important to activate the water molecules in your head, and they'll support you in performing the method. A clear conscious and focused mind with real intent is the key to jumping dimensions without any difficulty.

How Long Does It Take to Quantum Jump?

As you carefully follow the course of nature, you will observe a subtle yet very important thing. Nature always knows exactly how to provide the very best for mankind and does it selflessly. It doesn't however speed up its methods or processes for anyone. Everything is accomplished when the time is right and in perfect balance and harmony with the world. There needs to be equilibrium.

In the same way, you should have the patience necessary to see the results of quantum jumping. Do not rush and expect the results to appear immediately. All good things happen slowly. Even the tortoise won the race because it was calm, composed, slow, and steady.

Your desperation to see the results can alter your intentions and the procedure will not bring you any positive results. You need to follow the method carefully and patiently. It takes about 15 minutes, and then over time, the results begin to show. In the beginning, you need to visualize your desired results daily for two to three minutes.

It will help you tremendously if you develop a connection with the universe, a higher power, soul of the universe, or whatever you believe in. Having a spiritual relationship can help you tremendously. It will help you draw some serenity and composure, and also boost the positivity in your intentions. Any fear, anxiety, anger, or hesitation evaporates and the purity remains intact in your mind and soul.

Is It Harmful?

It is an absolutely safe method, and it will help you develop a better understanding of yourself. When you channel your intentions and think of all the good things in the world, the energy that you are drawing to yourself will either help you jump dimensions, or it will keep you exactly where you are. Whichever way, there is no physical or mental harm that can come to you that you could label as harmful or dangerous.

By attempting any of these exercises, you will either achieve what you set out to achieve or you won't. There's nothing to lose apart from possibly some time that it will take to complete either of these exercises.

What Can I Aim for During Quantum Jumping?

You can aim for absolutely anything you want, and that's the whole point of it. You can jump to any version of yourself that you would like. You can boost your health, stamina, productivity, emotional well-being, and wealth. Whatever you can truly imagine, whatever your heart desires. However, it is imperative that you keep the intention clear and do not overcrowd your mind with too many of them.

If you want to gain well-being, then focus only on your well-being. If you want to gain wealth, then focus only on wealth. With quantum jumping you don't need to acquire all the changes with your first attempt. You can repeat the same method over time to gain multiple benefits. Focus on only one particular thing that you would like to change during your first attempt.

How Do I Know if I Want to Quantum Jump?

If you are currently looking for new talents, or wish to be a better version of yourself than you are at present, then quantum jumping is for you. Whatever you seek, whether it is to improve any area in your life, find love, heal, get rid of ill-health, gain positivity, or gaining success, can all be achieved. You can consider this as a method of therapy as well. In the event that you are unhappy, anxious with the way your lifestyle is, or specific situations in your life are, you can choose to jump to a different dimension. You can be a better version of yourself and acquire that happiness and mental peace that you so desperately crave.

Summary

In this chapter, we have discussed that quantum jumping is something that is completely safe, natural, with no side effects. It can be performed by anyone as a means for them to gain whatever they want out of life. There are numerous multiverses with as many different versions of ourselves that we are able to tap into across space and distance by using water.

The entire process takes only 15 minutes to complete and you are free to repeat the process as often as you would like. It is important that you do not overcrowd your mind with too many things at once. When you are first beginning to attempt quantum jumping, focus on something small that you would like to change about yourself or in your life. You will really only be able to ascertain whether quantum jumping is for you or not once you have actually attempted it for yourself.

Your altered reality, or new future will not materialize overnight. You need to remember to be patient, trusting that the multiverse knows what it is doing and is in control.

Chapter 7: Understanding a Quantum Jumping

This concept was first introduced by Danish physicist Niels Bohr. His work in understanding how atomic particles are structured and laying the foundation for quantum theory earned him the Nobel Prize for Physics in 1922. Before you can understand this theory, you need to understand that we do not exist in a vacuum. There is matter all around us that fills up every single nook and cranny. What we think is space, consists of matter. The air around us consists of matter. Much of the matter that's in the air around us is actually water.

Matter consists of atoms, protons, electrons, which form molecules. Every single organism in the universe, or the multiverse, is made up of these molecules. This matter is sometimes referred to as cosmic soup. The reason for this is that even in the universe, matter and particles exist. It is not just an empty void of nothingness.

Charged molecules have been discovered by astrologers in the stars. While all this time we believe that we are the only inhabitants of this universe, these discoveries prove that all the molecular and chemical building blocks that we need to support life are in the universe already.

According to an astronomer from the National Radio Astronomy Observatory (NRAO) in Virginia, Tony Remijan, the discovery of these building blocks, as well as smaller organic molecules and amino acids, the universe has everything that it needs to support life on countless other planets (Reuland, 2007).

The definition provided for a quantum jump is the sudden change of what is known as a quantum system, from one state to another. A quantum system includes (atoms, molecules, and an atomic nucleus). As each of these systems absorb energy, they can move between high energy points and low energy points. For this to happen, the shift in energy has to occur.

You can only refer to something as a quantum jump when these properties exist in the molecular structure. It has to occur in a quantum system and not a conventional state. The other major difference is that while other changes can take place with matter, it usually happens gradually over time. A quantum jump happens very quickly. During a quantum jump, energy can either be emitted or absorbed.

How do these molecules move from one state to another though? This is all thanks to quantum physics and the seven laws of the universe. You need to be able to understand them to understand and accept quantum physics.

In a more straightforward sense, think of quantum jumping as re-tuning the radio or the frequency. There are many channels broadcasted at various frequencies. At your current frequency you might be emotionally unstable, overweight, or unhappy. All you have to do is tune in to a new frequency where you are happy, emotionally stable, and at a healthy weight. As part of the law of the universe, or the multiverse, be sure that you're not so focused on the past that this is what you are currently bringing into the present.

The words we choose all have power. When we focus on saying negative things while possibly complaining about our present state, the universe or multiverse may only hear what we are saying. As in the Law of Attraction, whatever we decide to "put out there," we need to accept that the universe/multiverse has absolutely no reason not to respond. It will give us whatever we are focusing on most of the time. For this purpose, we need to watch our thoughts, words, and actions. Whatever we focus on, the multiverse is only too happy to deliver.

You must know and believe that there are these alternate versions of you and a universe where these things are present. You are fit and happy in another dimension, and by shifting your consciousness, you can achieve that. That is what quantum jumping is. Over time you will see your health getting better, you will lose weight, and be more emotionally stable, and that is when you will have completely transitioned into this new dimension.

How Does This Technique Work?

Quantum jumping is a scientific technique that has a transforming effect on our lives. When we channel our energies with good intention focused towards a certain goal, our minds and bodies start to get tuned. The atoms in our body will start to align themselves such that they do actions and perform activities that work towards our goals. It's not just the intention that is going to bring about the change. You will consciously and subconsciously do things that will take you closer to your goal. Assuming that you want to lose weight, you will start exercising or going on a healthy diet without complaints. If you want to be rich, you will start working hard to earn the pennies that you want to see in your bank account. You will be energized with so much positive energy that your activities won't tire you or make you complain.

To understand the science behind quantum jumping, it is crucial that we understand some concepts. Though we are all aware of these from our school studies, we will be looking at them from the perspective of quantum jumping. Here are a few concepts that are vital to be understood.

The Law of Vibration - An In-Depth Look

The Law of Vibration is based on the fact that everything that exists in the universe, visible or invisible to the human eye, vibrates continuously at a particular frequency. Nothing in the universe rests. Even a solid material consists of small packets of energy that vibrate at a specific frequency. If we were to dissect anything in the universe at a quantum level, we would find that the core energy is the same in everything. Everything, from our thoughts to physical matter, is threaded with the same energy. At a subatomic level, we are all similar, and the same energy flows through all creations. You can call this energy the divine energy, soul of the universe, or the creative electric field.

Our thoughts, feelings, and intentions also carry vibrational energy, which is why our thoughts constantly keep emitting a particular vibration to the universe. Did you ever hear people say that they are getting negative vibes or that they are getting good vibes from a person? How do you think someone can feel these vibrations from the others? They can feel this because of the frequency emitting from the body of a person based upon their thoughts and emotions. It defines the kind of memories, ideas, and behaviors we have.

Thus, whatever resonates with our current frequency becomes our state of being. If you have had a rough couple of years, then it is possible that you are putting out unhappy thoughts or frequencies. The best part, however, is that no matter how many years it has been or how long you have lived in an unfortunate state, you can change your frequency in just a few minutes. It is as simple as turning on a switch. You can tune in to a higher desired form of vibration just by altering your consciousness.

Our thoughts create our reality. When we believe in a particular thought, it gets embedded in our subconscious and thus constantly emits a vibration with which our reality is shaped. We've already talked about the fact that 75% of our brain is water. Our brain consisting of 75% water means it can quickly respond to the changes in frequency, thoughts, and emotions. Water is highly receptive to everything around it, and so are we. Many consider the universe as the mind through which consciousness comes into existence.

Thus, by understanding the law of vibration, we

know that we all have the same energy within us and we all vibrate at a particular frequency. We are in the universe, and the universe is within us. Nothing we seek is different or separated from us. In our current state too, we exist in harmony with the universe, we just haven't transitioned our consciousness. Once we visualize our desired state, we can quickly make the shift to the new dimension.

The Double-Slit Experiment and Quantum Jumping

The critical experiment in the world of quantum physics is the double-slit experiment. It proves that quantum particles have a distinct nature to them. The experiment demonstrates that quantum particles behave in a specific way. They exhibit a wave-like motion. The very act of observing this experiment changes the way these quantum particles behave. It is entirely out of the box that quantum particles can even perceive that they are being watched and alter their behavior. Strange as this may seem, this is the key to the quantum world. The act of observing these particles alters their behavior dramatically.

Step 1: Solid Matter

To understand this experiment, imagine there's a wall directly in front of you with two holes or slits in it. You are standing on one side of the wall with a bucket of golf balls. As you begin throwing each of the golf balls at the wall several will bounce back to your side of the wall, while others will travel to the other side of the wall through one of the two slits. Now, what would happen if there was another wall behind the first? As each golf ball traveled through one of the slits it would in all likelihood end up hitting the second wall, not so.

Step 1: The Results

If you happened to be using golf balls covered with a form dye or dust that could actually mark the second wall as they struck, what do you suppose you would see? If you answered that you would see markings on the second wall that corresponded with the size and shape of each of the slits in the front wall, then you would be quite correct.

This is just the first step in this experiment.

Step 2: Light Waves

For the next step we are going to shine a colored light through each of the slits. For this experiment the distance between the slits needs to be approximately the same distance as the wavelength of the light. Light reacts completely differently from what our solid matter "golf balls" do. Instead of hitting the wall, the light actually splits into two separate waves. Similar to vibrations, each of these waves has an impact on the other.

Step 2: The Results

What you see as a result of this experiment is way different from the first. Here the light resembles water ripples when a pebble has been dropped into a mass of water. Depending on how the light is affected it reacts differently. In some instances, it can cancel itself out, while in other instances it forms what are known as peaks and troughs (or highs and lows). Where one peak meets another peak, the light waves are reinforced becoming stronger. This will result in the light becoming even brighter than what was initially shone through the slits. If these light waves are strong enough, they will create what's known as an inference pattern on the back wall. These are striped and result from the strengthened waves.

Step 3: Electrons

Taking this experiment even one step further. Let's move over to the quantum field.

Let's repeat the first experiment with the double slits. This time we are going to use electrons instead of golf balls. At the beginning of the experiment, seal off one of the slits and only fire the electrons through the first slit. This results in exactly what we saw with the golf balls, some of the electrons pass through and form the singular pattern of the slit in the wall that they passed through. Open the second slit and begin the process again, still using electrons.

Step 3: The Results

The result of this experiment however is going to prove to be completely different from what we would have expected. You would expect the electrons to respond exactly the same way as the golf balls did; after all, that's what passing through the single slit showed you. Not so fast, though. What has actually happened with the electrons is that there is an identical inference pattern which is what we saw when light waves passed through the double slits. This is pretty amazing, don't you think?

While this is pretty amazing, what can we learn from these three experiments?

This is what's so awesome about quantum physics is trying to figure out how these particles work. So, there are two separate hypotheses surrounding the reaction that the electrons had.

Step 3: Hypotheses

The first is that the electrons work similarly to light waves by interfering with one another. This would result in each particle hitting in a different place and at different times. The problem with this theory is that the same pattern holds even when firing these electrons one at a time. This discredits the theory that they're interfered with. What was noticed however is that every single dot made by an electron created a wave-like pattern.

The second hypothesis is that there's a splitting process that happens (also similar to light waves). This would infer that electrons then pass through both slits at the same time, interferes with itself, and somehow returns to its original form hitting the back wall as a single unit.

Step 3: Under Observation

In trying to prove the above hypotheses a detection device was placed in each of the slits to try and measure the exact behavior of these particles.

The result? Suddenly the particles decide to behave and represent the two perfectly formed lines as we had in our golf ball experiment. It was as if the particles were able to somehow "comprehend" that they were being monitored and decided to react completely differently.

What Can Be Learned From These Experiments?

From a quantum physics perspective, what we refer to as electrons or particles display dual characteristics. They display characteristics of waves, as well as reacting completely differently when being observed. Here they behaved like solid matter (golf balls). This provides a bit of a conundrum for quantum mechanics as nobody is quite certain why this occurs (Marianne, 2020).

Why the Double-Slit Experiment Is So Important

The critical experiment in the world of quantum physics is the double-slit experiment. It proves that quantum particles have a probabilistic nature. It is demonstrated that the quantum particles exhibit a wave function and the act of observation changes the way they behave. It is entirely out of the box that quantum particles can even perceive that they are being watched and alter their behavior. Strangely, this is the key to the quantum world.

The universe is an ocean of quantum particles which has a wave function of probability and possibility. It is only through the consciousness that the outcomes are streamlined for us. Our awareness affects our reality at a fundamental level. It is what governs our reality.

There are a million possibilities and probabilities in the universe, but the moment we think of something or believe it to be true, it manifests. It is essential to keep in mind that there are a vast number of possibilities and they all can come true only if you believe in them.

Another important factor here is the act of observing. The intent and the consciousness of the observer can make or break the experiment. The result of the experiment entirely depends upon the mindset of the observer. If the intention to jump and the desired outcome is communicated clearly, then you will be able to jump the dimensions easily. The result of the experiment entirely depends upon you. As mentioned above, it is your consciousness that streamlines the probability and possibilities in the universe. It is through your mindset that your reality manifests. That is what the quantum double-slit experiment has taught us. Let's now move to the theory of quantum entanglement and its role in quantum jumping.

Quantum Entanglement

This phenomenon tells us that two quantum particles share a relationship which is independent of time and space. A simple example would be that no matter where these two quantum particles are in time and space, if one turns clockwise the other will turn anticlockwise. It is peculiar because the quantum particles are not physically in contact. However, the energy that is within and around the quantum particles is responsible for their relationship. That is how these quantum particles can communicate, travel, and jump from one dimension to another.

Quantum entanglement happens when these particles actually connect with one another and then act in exactly the same way, but only when they're being observed. There are rules in quantum physics that confirm these photons are all around us all the time. They can take on various states simultaneously. Now, here's what Albert Einstein called "spooky action at a distance," if they are observed or physically measured they spin. This spin looks like it is rotational, but pairs of particles are actually interacting with one another.

This happens over time and distance, which is what makes it relevant to quantum jumping. What happens in place A with the particles, also happens in place B (potentially hundreds or even thousands of miles away). The movement that is observed causes light refraction and both photons are transferring energy at 10,000 times the speed of light.

The first images of proof of quantum entanglement have been published by physicists at the University of Glasgow, Scotland. It actually shows how particles react in a mirror-image to one another over distance, proving that they are linked to one another. numerous experiments were conducted, resulting in four separate images of entangled particles as they transitioned through four different phases (MacDonald, 2019).

When you perform the quantum jumping technique, the quantum particles are able to communicate, interact with each other, and make the quantum leap possible. Each element of your body consists of the same quantum particles as that of the water and the universe. So, once the desired outcome is communicated clearly to the water and universe, each cell in your body can copy the same intention and perform the quantum jump. That is how quantum entanglement plays its role. I hope as we move from one concept to another you are gaining a better understanding.

Water and Its Importance in This Method

You are familiar by now with the miraculous and unique abilities of water. As we just read in the section above about quantum entanglement, the same quantum particles exist in water as they exist in the universe. We know that water is capable of understanding our emotions, feelings, and intent. Not only does the water understand, but it also reacts and can memorize the same emotions and intent. When we communicate our current state to the water, it entraps that vibration which we are on.

The moment we express our desired state to the water, its frequency shifts. The quantum particles in the water begin to alter their frequency due to the transition in your consciousness. When we drink the water, we are in the state of transition, and the water helps in communicating the same message to every cell it comes in contact with. After all, more than 60% of our body is water.

We have already read that water responds to various thoughts, captures memory, and it can replicate a similar molecular structure as is shown to it. If one drop of Zamzam water can turn 1000 ml of water into Zamzam water, then I believe the water can help us in shifting our frequency and in jumping dimensions.

Summary

In this chapter, we have covered various scientific and physic laws and information, as well as experiments that still leave scientists scratching their heads. The Double-Slit Experiment also proves that molecules behave differently when they're being observed, proving that they have a level of consciousness. They are aware of being observed and change their behavior entirely.

We have also learned the meaning of quantum entanglement and why water is so important for us to know how to use it to our best advantage. Given the amount of power and energy that is stored in water, we have the exact same power available to us. It has been confirmed that if we could lay each molecule of water that we each have in our bodies side to side, or end to end, there are enough of them to reach all the way around the globe. Surely this must change the way you think about water as it flows throughout your body? Not only that, but we have the potential to harness the energy contained in all the H2O in our bodies.

Chapter 8:
How to Perform the Two-Glass Method for Quantum Jumping

Now that you know the mechanism of how quantum jumping happens and why water is an integral part of performing the two-glass method, you will be able to perform it efficiently. Follow the step-by-step guide outlined below to perform the method. I will urge you to finish reading the book first and then return to this page when you decide to take the leap. It will give you a profound understanding of water, quantum jumping, divine power, and oneness. So, let's begin!

Intentions You Should Hold While Performing the Two-Glass Method

It is imperative that the intention is vivid and defined. When you decide to shift from your current state to the desired state, the visualization should be as real as possible. Try to imagine yourself in the desired state and living in that moment. Don't think of it as a distant dream. Instead, try to experience it through your consciousness. Doing so will begin the frequency transition and the same will be communicated to the water at a molecular level.

Apart from the clear and vivid visualization, it is essential to link the transition to God, the universe, divine power, or the ultimate source of energy. You can call it whatever you want, but associating the change with the ultimate power will positively affect the method.

When you associate the jumping method to God, or whatever higher power you choose to revere, you also seek the approval of the universe. You are no longer the sole observer of your transition. Divine love, gratitude, and positive feelings will grow in your heart because you are performing the method by remembering the divine power. It will cause you to have pure and stronger emotions, consciousness, and all of this will lead to a positive outcome.

Moreover, combining your intention with God will enrich your heart with gratitude. Once we declare that we want to achieve the outcome via God's will and not ours, there is no room for any negative feeling. If we do it with our intention alone, we might give ourselves credit which may lead to ego and other negative emotions. That is why you must always remember your higher power and offer your gratitude after you have completed the method.

Even after you have completed the method, you must try to re-visualize the same feelings while remembering the divine power. It is essential to keep in contact with the divine power and to keep the desired state in mind. Remember the divine power with gratitude and love, after you manifest the desired state. It will help you to live your life in a total state of well-being further.

When Should You Perform the Two-Glass Method?

The best time of the day to perform this method of quantum jumping is either early in the morning or late in the evening, preferably before you go to bed, or after you wake up in the morning. There's a specific reason for this. It is during this time of the day that your subconscious mind has the greatest control over your body. Although your conscious mind is awake, it is not fully alert and at the forefront of our reasoning just yet. That spot is held by the subconscious.

The subconscious is more alert and energized than the conscious mind. By now we realize that we need the power of our subconscious mind to achieve quantum jumping. Throughout the rest of the day, the conscious mind will be overstimulated, hyperactive, giving you less time to focus, think, or meditate. You are programmed to work mechanically and do what you do every day.

Routine is what makes your conscious mind stronger while your subconscious remains calm in the background. You must practice this method at a time when you are in a calm, and stress-free state. This will help you numb your anxious, conscious mind and open new doors where you can see new possibilities. You will acquire a better perspective because of the subconscious mind that holds more information, emotions, thoughts, ideas, and theories that remain hidden during a stressful day. Practicing it in the morning or late at night will allow you to concentrate better, you will be able to visualize what you want, and be able to control your mind.

The Two-Glass Method

Few people associate the two-glass method of quantum jumping with the law of attraction. While it may sound like it is difficult to do it is quite the opposite. This method is easy to use. All that you need is two clear glasses, two pieces of paper (post-it notes are ideal), something to attach the paper to each glass, and a pen.

The Method

The first glass represents the current reality that you

are experiencing, while the second glass represents a future state or reality that you would like to experience. These two states are physically connected by the vibrationally charged energy contained in the water.

Using the first post-it note or piece of paper, capture your current reality. What are you experiencing currently in your life? This could be anything from relationship problems, to being desperately unhappy in your current position at work. Maybe you feel that you deserve a raise or a promotion that you have applied for? Whatever you may presently be unhappy with in your life, or you wish you could change. Do not worry about how long the list is. If you have used a large sheet of paper (letter size), fold it until it is about the same size as a conventional post-it note so it is easy to attach to the glass. When you are finished with this list, attach it to the full glass of water.

Now, taking the second piece of paper, write down everything that you would like to experience in your reality instead. Be careful when it comes to the words that you use throughout this process. Remember that our thoughts and words hold intention and whatever we are currently thinking is what will come back to us. Consider each of the experiments we have conducted in the chapters above, as well as all the work done by Dr. Emoto. He proved that even intention can be held by water.

If you want that promotion, write it down. You want to rekindle that relationship, write it down, in the present tense as if it has already happened. Avoid using any negative words. The universe and multiverse cannot distinguish between good and bad. It will hear and respond to what you are asking for. If you want wealth, ask for it. Health; ask for it. Love; ask for it. If you are presently suffering from an illness or disease, thank God, the divine power, the universe, or whoever you choose to worship for granting you the desires of your heart. However, always ensure that the intention is in keeping with the will of the creator of the universe and the multiverse and not according to your own will.

Fold this paper and attach it to the empty glass. Before attaching each piece of paper to each glass consider the differences between the two lists (this is why post-it notes are a better option, you can consider them each alongside one another on each glass).

Begin the process of pouring the water from the full glass into the empty glass. You can use mindfulness techniques as you do so by focusing entirely on the water as it slowly flows from the full glass to the empty glass. Watch the movement of the water, paying close attention to the shapes that it makes. What does the water sound like as it is flowing from the one glass into the other?

While this is happening, focus on the things that you want and are asking for. Imagine how good it will feel when they materialize in your reality. How will you feel about your additional wealth? How will you feel when you are in that special new relationship? How will you feel when your boss announces your new promotion?

Having completed the transference of the water from your present reality glass, to your future reality glass, slowly drink the water from the second glass. Hold in your mind that what you wrote down on the second piece of paper, your intention, is now your reality. We have spoken of vibrations and how important they are when it comes to sending out our message to the multiverse. Hold in your mind the intention that this is now your reality.

When you have finished drinking this glass of water, say thank you to the multiverse. You can now continue with your normal routine.

It is important to work alongside the universe and the multiverse to be sure that these things happen for you in your life. If you want a brand-new relationship with someone, be on the lookout for this special person. Place yourself in situations where you are likely to meet the kind of person you are hoping to meet. It does not help to anticipate a promotion at work unless you physically apply for one. Nothing in the universe happens by chance, there needs to be some form of action that takes place on our part for the universe to respond positively to your requests.

Intention is something that is genuine, and very powerful. Remember that everything that you put out into the universe has vibrational energy and the universe responds. Your vibrational energy needs to be as high as possible for your desires to be manifest. The highest vibration is that of love. Express your love for everything you already have, as well as those things you know will manifest in your life. Live your life as though you have already received these things, or they are already on their way to you.

Finally, give thanks to the universe for providing you with your new reality. You should begin to believe that this is now so and live your life as though you are in possession of your intentions. Wishing for something will not make it come to pass in your present reality. You need to appreciate that you now need to get out there to make things happen. There will be no change or shift taking place unless you do everything necessary to believe that a shift is happening, and you are one with the creator for your new reality.

Time and Place

Set aside sufficient time for you to be able to practice this technique daily, or weekly, as often as you feel the need. The best time is either early morning or late at night, as explained in the previous sections. You need to be comfortable in the space that you choose. It should be quiet, and free from any and all distractions. If you meditate by practicing yoga, chanting, or any other creative task in the space you have chosen then this will be an ideal spot for you.

Find a place where you will feel closer to yourself, confident, happy, and at one with the universe. It is very important to let friends, family, and children know that this is your private time and you are not to be disturbed or interfere with your routine. You should feel peaceful and calm in the space, almost as if it were sacred to you. It must be your own personal paradise where there is no place for negativity.

Minimize Distractions

Reduce the electromagnetic signals in the area. Switch off your wireless internet modem (Wi-Fi) as well as your smartphone, laptop, unplug anything that draws current within the area so that you don't experience any electromagnetic disturbances. Other household items include the TV, microwave, and other electronic devices in the house. You are trying to avoid transference of any electrical charge being transferred to the water.

Anything that potentially can hold a charge should be turned off. In the experiment with Luc Montagnier, they needed to switch off all bright lights, spotlights, and recording equipment so that radio waves and frequency were not transferred to corrupting the experiment. Be keenly aware of your thoughts during this process. You want to have only the best feelings and intentions so that the water can respond to the vibrations that you can emit simply with an intention. Be sure that your thoughts are focused totally on this routine and that you're not distracted by other things unnecessarily.

Before You Begin

Prepare a rough draft of what you want to write on each of the sheets of paper. You need to think carefully about what you want to write for your current state, as well as the desired state. Keep your words to a minimum. Take your time to consider all the things that you would really like to change in your current reality and how you would like your future reality to be. Think about the words that you are going to write, remember that words themselves hold tremendous power.

Consider the laws of polarity and how writing one thing may possibly attract the exact opposite. Think about each of the frequencies that these words are likely to move you to. An excellent example of this might be a desire to change your current work, or your career. Write on the paper for your current state: current - unfulfilling job, desired - a fulfilling job. By keeping your words to a minimum, your message is delivered to the universe and easily understood by the universe. Remember the acronym: K. I. S. S. (keep in short and simple).

Think About What You Want to Do

Once you've prepared a draft version of what you want to write and change, examine yourself deeply and think of things you are not happy with currently at your job (or whatever situation you are trying to change). Set a clear intention backed with strong emotions as to why you want to shift to the desired state. In this particular case, one can think about how dreams are not being fulfilled at work professionally and financially.

It could be anything from your current workload, a dominating boss, an unpleasant atmosphere in the office with co-workers. You may be totally unmotivated in the work that you're doing. You may believe that you deserve more than what you are rewarded with for the talent that you possess. You may find that the commute to and from work every day is simply becoming too pressurized.

Try to bring in the sense of unfulfillment due to less salary, a non-rewarding position, or lack of opportunities to grow and learn. Assign these thoughts with real feelings. When your mind is clear, you can sit down to begin the process.

While we have briefly run through the process above, we will now go over a detailed step-by-step approach that you are able to follow. Remember to read to the end of this book and then return to this page before attempting any quantum jumps.

Start the Method

Sit comfortably and think of God, Allah, or the divine power of the universe and ask for its presence and blessing for the method you are about to perform. This will help to neutralize any negative feelings, strengthen your consciousness and open your mind to peace and enlightenment. A very important part of this process is for your vibrational energy to be in the right place from the beginning. This is where you need to be focusing on this energy.

Think About What You Want to Change and Write It Down

Each of the two pieces of paper should have two different headings. The first should be the current state, and the second, the desired state. You can refer to your rough draft that you put together for the things that you'd like to see change in your life, as well as those things you would like to see materialize in your life.

Write down your list of things that you want to change in regards to your current state and what you would like to experience in your desired state. Keep each list short, to the point, and in simple language. Remember that the universe will give you whatever you ask of it, but you need to understand how to do so without making it confusing. Keep each of your glasses separate and attach one of the notes to each of the glasses. What is vitally important at this point is that the glasses don't get mixed up, and you remain clear as to which glass is which.

Pour Water Into the Current State Glass

Add clean, fresh water to the current state glass. Try and find water that is as close to natural spring water as possible, but it should definitely be safe enough for drinking. All water retains memory of everything it has either come into contact with or been exposed to. For this reason it's better to consider pure spring water, preferably bottled at the source in glass bottles (remember about the BPA).

Your goal is to find water that has as few contaminants as possible. We spoke earlier about how water is piped by thousands of kilometers of piping with bends and twists. By the time you turn your tap on, those water molecules are what can be referred to as "angry." Who can blame them - they have been bounced around bashing sharp pipes, corners, and bends for goodness knows how long. This water is not ideal for completing the two-glass method, unless you are somehow able to purify it first by blessing it. Angry water will have angry memories attached to it.

Current State

Hold the current state glass in your hands and look at the water. Begin to visualize your current situation, the state that you find yourself in, and attach the feelings that you feel while looking at the water. There are two ways of doing this effectively and there is no right or wrong way. You can either think each of these thoughts or speak them out loud while looking at the water. Allow your strongest emotions to take over, and let the universe know how bad you feel or are affected by the current state. Be sure that your intentions are clear and that the universe can understand your communication.

Forgiveness and Love

Set your intentions to the water, apologizing for anything that you may have done wrong and ask the water for forgiveness and love after you communicate the current state. Being able to forgive yourself for being in that state and offer yourself love to heal from the pain of unfulfillment. Should there be someone that you're holding a grudge against, forgive that person as well. In this example, you should excuse your boss and the employees who possibly trouble you in the workplace. Excuse the system at work that is preventing you from growing.

Take your time to forgive yourself, your circumstances in your present state and offer love to both. Doing so will help you to forgive yourself, your circumstances, and offer love to both. This will help you heal and will also get rid of any negative vibrations. Often we hold grudges against people and ourselves, and these feelings will prevent a person from quantum jumping. Therefore, it is better to forgive yourself, others, and offer gratitude that you are getting rid of the situation.

It is important that you forgive your parents, friends, family, or anyone else who was a participant or a contributor to the current state. The person making the quantum leap is the same; therefore, it is necessary to get rid of any baggage that might exist in this state. If you try to jump with unresolved feelings, these feelings might travel with you, or may not lead to a successful shift in the dimension. For this reason it's important to forgive yourself and offer yourself love. (Love also operates at the highest possible vibrational frequency).

Place the Current State Cup Down

It is now time for you to pour the water from the current state glass to the desired state glass. This should not be rushed because it should be done with intention. While pouring the water, think about God, Allah, the divine power, or the universe, and seek its blessing to begin the transition.

Desired State

When you have poured the water into the desired state glass, hold it again in both hands. Stare at the water while visualizing what you want to achieve. Try and feel accomplished, fulfilled, and happy as if it were real.

Harness positive emotions and the vivid details of your desired state.

For example, the job role, the office, the salary, clothes you would wear, things you would do in the office, the lifestyle you would have, the rewards you would get, the happiness you would feel, the sense of accomplishment you would attain and other such emotions. This will help create a compelling visualization.

Bless the Water

Once again, bless the water, asking it to help you reach your desired state. When you have finished communicating the desired state to the water, lift the cup and drink the water while envisaging that the water is helping you achieve all that you want to achieve. Feel the water flow through your mouth, down your esophagus, and then settling in your stomach. Feel the frequency influence the cells in your body and relax your mind and body in response to it.

Place the Empty Cup Down and Thank the Divine Power

Express your gratitude toward Him for providing you with the resources and thank Him in advance for what you are about to receive from the universe.

Once you have completed this method, try to go to

sleep or sit quietly for some time. For the next few days, try to remember the divine power and imagine the desired state. This will help you transition and accept the outcome. Moreover, it will assist in building a spiritual connection with the omniscient energy. This does not mean that you will focus all your energies on thinking about that piece of paper and your quantum jumping method.

Keep these thoughts in your mind, but also work and continue with your daily routine. A lazy person with fantasies will not achieve their goals unless they gear up and do something to change the course of their life. Believe that the multiverses are supporting you in your efforts and draw the energy from the divine source to take steps toward a different dimension.

If you perform the method this way, it will help in a successful quantum jumping experience. You will begin to see results within a few days. It could be the slightest or most significant sign based on how you performed the method. Ultimately, the consciousness and the visualization by the individual performing the jump will determine the outcome. therefore, try and avoid any negativity, distractions, and above all, believe in the possibilities of the universe.

Your belief system is stronger than you think. Once you start to envision yourself in a particular state, you also need to believe that you are capable of achieving that. And that's how it should be. You must believe that you deserve all those great things before you achieve them.

Self-doubt is a dangerous thing and slowly allows negativity and loss to creep into your life. Each of us is sent into this world with the same potential. But, what makes each of us different is our ability to tap into that potential, believe in our strength, and ultimately do what we are meant to do. Love yourself and pamper yourself in the same way that you would do with anyone else you love. Put yourself at the top of your list of priorities, and do not let negativity spoil your enthusiasm.

Quantum jumping will open new doors for you. Shift from your hut to the tall mansion. Leave your dirty clothes behind, and dress yourself in the best clothes from Zara. Stop eating unhealthy food and only accept juicy, fresh, and beneficial fruits and vegetables. Do not hate yourself for being obese, and believe that you can cut the fat with a silver sword.

Be happy about jumping dimensions and accept that the change is doing you good. Our mind is like unexplored territory. It's a bit like Narnia, and you are the lion who rules what happens there. Hold all the power in your hands, take the help of water and dimensions to achieve whatever you want. Put all excuses behind you and imagine yourself to be the King or Queen of your own world. At the end of the day, you are what you believe yourself to be. Give yourself the best status that you deserve. Happy living

I hope you have understood the mechanism behind the two-cup method and that it does not come across as some hogwash based on scientific facts only. Now let me offer you the step by step method of how to perform the quantum jumping technique.

Summary

This entire chapter has been devoted to mastering the two-glass method of quantum jumping. As promised, you can see how simple and straightforward this experience can be. It is important to follow each instruction to the letter. While some things happen more quickly than others, you will notice that there will be times when you can immediately feel a major shift taking place in your life. If this is so, you know that you are now becoming an expert at this brand-new form of attracting whatever you want into your life.

If things are not materializing as quickly as you had hoped, there may be several things that you are possibly doing wrong. The first is being too vague about what you want. You may be expecting things to happen too quickly, without doing any of the work yourself. You may be sending conflicting signals because your emotions are all over the place. Remember that water reacts to emotions quite radically. I can literally go on and on with things you may be doing wrong.

As suggested, read till the end of the book before attempting either of these methods and only then return to see what mistake(s) you made and when.

Chapter 9:
The One-Glass Method

So far we have taken a look at the two-glass method used to quantum jump. While this is the more well-known method of using water to jump, it's not the only method that can be used. The one-glass method is similar to the two-glass method, only as you can see by its name, we use one glass instead of two. Not only this, but the method requires you to both manifest and envision the life you want while channeling your energy into the water you're going to use for your quantum jump.

I know what you're thinking. Channeling my energy? Well, if you believe that both the current universe and the multiverse are made up of energy, then you'll understand what I mean by channeling your energy.

As an entity of Earth, in your current universe, you

can harness energy. What you think becomes reality and your very ability to read or go for a walk requires energy input, like when you eat food for instance. Throughout the universe everything is made up of and connected by energy. One force pulls while the other pushes, and it is this energy within ourselves that creates the link or channel between us and the multiverse version of yourself. Because we are the same thing existing at the same time, only in a different dimension or universe, our energies can easily connect.

Since we now know that water is a conductor and storer of energy, it creates the perfect receptacle to pick up vibrations that are traveling across the universe, multiverse, and dimension to reach you in your current state. Vibrations are sent back and forth between you and your multiverse itself. These vibrations are picked up by the water in your body. Waves travel through water much quicker than in air due to its density and can therefore channel multiverses much quicker and more efficiently.

Perhaps you're thinking, why would I need two different methods that should have the same outcome? Well, the one-glass method is slightly different because of the way it is performed and the reason it's being performed. This method is mostly aimed at fixing things you are not happy with, things that you have absolutely no control over. This chapter is going to take a look at what you need, how to perform the one-glass method, and how to keep positive while everything you've channeled starts to come true.

What Is the One-Glass Method?

There are several differences between the two-glass method and the one-glass method. While at the same time there are various similarities. With both methods you are going to write down your intention so you can send this into the universe or the multiverse to achieve whatever you want out of life. One of the main differences when using the single glass method is that obviously you are only using one glass of water.

It should be noted that this doesn't make this process any less effective because you are only using one glass. There are several other differences when it comes to the one-glass method which you should pay close attention to so you know what to do. Once again, it is best to finish reading through this book before attempting any of these quantum jumps.

This method is very powerful when it comes to manifestation and is often used when the person is looking to change something that is completely out of their control. By this I mean things that you cannot actively change yourself, such as how someone else feels. Think of it as a type of persuasion tool; you manifest better outcomes for yourself by envisioning the outcome you'd prefer. Pretty amazing don't you think?

I'm sure you're still wondering if, or even how, all of this really works. I mean, how can water and quantum jumping manifest a better life? Just remember that everything in our world is connected and it is further connected to the universe, and our universe is then connected to the multiverse. It is this link between everything that allows us to channel into these connections.

It may seem as though both methods are almost exactly the same, but the one-glass method needs the direct input of your own energy in your current universe or state, only. The direct input of your own energy can be seen as what connects you, the channel that connects your current frequency to the multiple versions of you across the multiverse. Almost like when you watch TV, the image travels along in waves (your energy frequency and the water) and finally reaches the receiver (you and the water) and projects an image (your wishes coming true). Your mind is used as the projector or TV screen to see your other self in order to learn from them or ask questions that may aid your current state in whatever you're asking for.

Similarly, you will need to write down what it is that you **cannot** control in your current universe, such as a health issue or maybe even a lost lover. The idea is that your energies between you and your multiple selves amplify the vibrations through your connection. Now you place the glass of water on top of your wish, and you're ready to begin tapping into this simple method of quantum jumping.

What You'll Need

This method is very simple and I can guarantee that most if not all readers will have the equipment needed to perform this method. For the one-glass method, you will need four things, five if you count yourself. Get yourself a glass from the kitchen, some clean, fresh water, and a pen and paper. If you don't have a glass you can use a cup, but glass is always better to use because of its ability to resonate energy. This means that the glass can pick up vibrations that are being sent out.

That is why using it to channel energy from the multiverse is ideal. It amplifies the experience because it amplifies the connection between you and your multiverse self. Once again, the reason for using clear glass is because it is made of silica, or sand, which comes from the Earth, and is another natural element.

Find an area that you feel most connected to. It should be quiet and free of any distractions, much like the setting for the two-glass method. You can perform either method anywhere you feel the most comfortable, but keep in mind that the area you choose should have a positive feel to it, because this positive energy adds to the water's molecular structure that combines with the water currently present in your body and changes its molecular structure, too.

Areas that are great for positive energy input are areas in nature such as the garden or nature reserves. Even having spent time in nature before performing a quantum jump can improve the energy. Dr. Emoto strongly believed in the ability of water to heal people, and after discovering water's consciousness and ability to remember, it made sense to use water exposed to positivity to rectify the negativity in the sick.

As you remember from Chapter 3, I mentioned water's ability to store information and replicate the molecular structures it comes into contact with at any point. This memory is what allows the positive energy to change the water currently in your body to the same positive structure as the glass you've just consumed. The idea is to tap into the positive energy that allowed the successful versions of yourself to accomplish what you haven't been able to.

The One-Glass Method
Step 1: Your Desire(s)

We begin at the spot you've chosen to perform the method. Remember the pen and paper you need? Begin to write down the thing you want to change. Perhaps you and a friend aren't speaking anymore or you're hoping to get into the university you just applied to. Whatever it is that you want to change in your current universe, write it down on the page. If the page you used is a large one, fold it in half. Set the glass on the folded page and fill it with that water I mentioned. Now comes the fun part, the quantum jump.

Something that is extremely important in this method that is different from the first is that whatever you decide to write down needs to be written in the present tense. Avoid using words such as "I'd like to…" or "I want…" Instead, write your desires in the present tense. As though you are already in possession of your desires. Use words such as "I'm so happy now that …" or "I have enough … and am so grateful for …"

Remember that gratitude operates on a high vibration, similar to that of love. When you are at one with the universe, and the multiverse, and you express gratitude for the abundance that you have in your life, you are all the more likely to be given more. Like any typical parent, the universe is only too happy to reward a grateful child.

Step 2: Set Your Intention

Fold the page, or place the page under the full glass of water. Focus intently on exactly what you have written down and what you would like the universe to manifest for you in your life. This could be anything from health, happiness, wealth, career development, a new home, a new love interest, absolutely anything you can clearly visualize and believe you are worthy of can be yours to enjoy.

The water needs to be as pure as it can possibly be. If you know that your building has rusty old pipes, rather purchase pure spring water that says that it's bottled at the source and be certain that it's also in a glass bottle. Fill your glass almost to the brim with this clean, fresh, spring water.

Step 3: Energize Yourself

We've learned that heat can change the molecular structure of water and everything in the universe and multiverse operates on vibrations. So, what is the best way to create an environment for the water in your single glass? Without needing any fancy equipment or a laboratory, all you need is yourself.

Place the glass on top of the piece of paper where you have written what you would like to see manifest in your current life. This next part is great fun. You need to generate heat in the palms of your hands by rubbing them together fairly briskly. Once your hands are nice and warm, place your hands on either side of the glass by cupping your palms facing inwards toward the glass. Hold your hands about 1 inch away from the side of the glass on either side. The goal of this activity is for you to transfer your energy to the water.

Step 4: Visualize Your Future

As you are channeling this energy, focus on what you would like to have manifest. The image that you visualize in your head should be as clear as possible. These images should allow you to feel all the emotions associated with having, experiencing, becoming, whatever it is that you desire. All the while your hands should remain on either side of the glass. You are using your current universal energy as the portal to your other self in another universe and dimension.

Step 5: Return to the Present

After visualizing what you want and are you brought back or feel comfortable with coming back to your current universe, drink the water that is in the glass. Some like to drink from it throughout their day, while others will drink the entire glass after the quantum jump. This is up to you. As long as you drink the water until it is finished, what the water remembers will be transferred to you.

In the two-glass method, negativity is taken out of the water by cleaning it with positive thoughts before you transfer it to the glass that represents your desire or the circle of energy you allow in, while with the one-glass method it requires you to purify the water of ill or negativity by absorbing the energy around you to travel to your various selves across dimensions and the multiverse. The positive energy you witness when meeting your other self channels into your current state to begin rewarding you your vision.

Step 6: Go About Your Day

Don't think about it too much afterward. Most people, after they perform either method, expect their world to change the second the water hits their lips. Yes, it does begin to change from that very second, but big changes happen at a pace the universe knows you can handle. If everything was thrown at you all at once, you might struggle to juggle it all and it is for this reason that you should be patient after drinking the water. Keep the image of what you want in your head whenever you do think of it, but don't allow it to consume your every thought because then you won't see the changes unfolding before your eyes.

Am I Rich Yet?

Remember when I mentioned that you shouldn't obsess over your visualization? The reason you should allow yourself to continue as normal after doing either the one glass or two-glass method is that you won't be able to focus on the rest of your journey if you do. After performing either of these methods, remember to be thankful to your version of a higher power.

Thank it for allowing you to channel your energy

through the water and yourself to the other version of you in a parallel universe or dimension, and then only truly ponder on it when it enters your mind at random. Humans think constantly, both consciously and subconsciously.

To be able to keep your thoughts in line with the energy you channeled during your quantum jump, you need to keep your visualization alive and positive whenever it pops into your head. Don't allow it to be tainted with negative energy, because you are constantly sending this energy back and forth between this universe and the multiverse.

Channeling these thoughts are important, and it's not to say that you should never think of them, because the more you picture it the more it will manifest, but if it's all that you think about then you don't allow for the other good energies that are actually from you performing the method to take place.

Relax after doing your quantum jump, have a warm bath, or go out into the garden and think for a while about all the things you are grateful for, all the things you believe you deserve, and all the things you've done that have either helped or hindered your progress thus far. I have mentioned the important role that gratitude and love can have in this process. They are able to increase your vibrational energy substantially and this is what you need to see your dreams and desires manifest in your lives.

Summary

This chapter took a look at the other method that can be used for quantum water jumping, known as the one-glass method. It's similar to the two-glass method, but the focus is more on using your own energy to channel your jump while also solely focusing on changing things that almost seem impossible to change, like the attitude of a friend or someone's feelings towards you.

Even though this is a safe and easy way to make a better life for yourself, you must remind yourself not to obsess over those things that you want for yourself in the future. Don't forget who you are as things start to change for the better in your world. Take away from this chapter that water is powerful, and even more so when you use it to quantum jump for a better life, but don't get too caught up in your thoughts; otherwise, you won't be able to reap what you have sown, and that could be all that you could ever have asked for.

Conclusion

We live in a world that is forever changing. As human beings, we have been searching for answers to some of life's deepest questions since we learned how to speak. Being willing to open our minds to things that seem impossible has proven time and time again to deliver positive results in the lives of some of even the most skeptical of individuals.

Quantum jumping using water may not be for everybody, and that's okay. But those that have tried either or both of these methods to gain wealth, love, and even happiness will tell you that it works and they won't go back to what is considered the "norm" ever again.

The use of quantum jumping has resulted in many positive results for so many people, and has such a large following because of it. Those that have chosen quantum jumping, whether with water or not, have experienced great outcomes. Those that haven't used water before are beginning to understand the power that water holds and how it can actually increase the results exponentially when performing a jump.

Both the one and two-glass method can be performed by anyone. That's right, as long as you have a clear intention when performing either jump you will begin to see results. It makes them the ideal method for quantum jumping because of water's ability to remember, replicate, and store energy.

Channeling multiple universes and dimensions can take a lot of energy, and by allowing the positive energy from the universe and by allowing all that positive energy from the universe you are channeling to be stored in the water that you drink, you are changing the molecular structure of the water that is present in your body in your current universe.

The water retains the energy of your wishes and your desires. It duplicates the molecular structure of whatever it is that your parallel self has done to gain what you don't have, and by consuming the water you have added this constant back and forth frequency that takes from your parallel self's energy and adds to your energy in your current state.

It can often be quite scary to think of something as simple as water as being alive and able to give us all that we've ever desired. However, through the works of Dr. Masaru Emoto and the various scientific discoveries in the quantum physics field, it has been proven that water is not only necessary for life, but is alive itself.

If one looks at the way water functions in a natural setting such as a river or ocean, it can absorb and store large amounts of heat energy from the sun. Notice I said store. If one believes that everything is made up of energy, then the fact that water is able to hold onto it proves that the vibrations released when you quantum jump can be absorbed and stored in the water you use during either the one- or two-glass method.

To begin your journey of advanced quantum water jumping using water, you will need to open your mind completely and have an intention. Remember that your intention can be anything that your heart desires, but there are always consequences. Hoping for something bad to happen to someone or something else will create negative energy that can result in exactly the opposite of what you had envisioned for yourself.

Without following the fundamental guidelines which have been presented to you throughout this book, you will block your ability to manifest the best possible life for yourself. Negativity and skepticism vibrate on the same frequency as your positive energy, and too much negativity will, much like a radio signal, interfere with the signals you are sending out and warp them.

Remember that every action has an equal and opposite reaction. This is known as Newton's third law, and it can be applied throughout the current universe, as well as the multiverse. Now that you have filled yourself with the knowledge of using water for quantum jumping, go out and manifest your perfect reality, one glass of water at a time.

What to Take Away From These Experiences

It is very easy to get lost in a sea of conflicting beliefs and ideas which we happen to see in the world today, but quantum jumping and jumping using water are both safe and easy methods of manifestation that, as I've mentioned many times before, can be done by absolutely anyone that has an unwavering positive intention for a better life.

Understand that things will begin to change immediately, but because you are dealing with quantum physics, this doesn't mean you will notice every single change as and when it happens. You may start to notice a positive change in your mood, or maybe you get noticed at work, where before you went completely unnoticed.

Quantum jumping is very powerful and if you do it right you will begin to reap the rewards. If by chance you have only recently been introduced to quantum jumping, or using water to quantum jump and are still not sure, the best thing to do is to try. There is absolutely no harm in attempting something that has no negative side effects. I hope that you have found some valuable information in this book and begin to make use of quantum jumping and the miraculous properties of water to your advantage.

Make the most of every opportunity available to you to master these very powerful techniques using either of these two methods to receive everything that the universe and multiverse have to offer you. Begin today by setting powerful, positive intentions, absorbing all the energy that is rightfully yours. Improve the quality of your life both simply, and safely.

As an author, it is always my intention to deliver information that is informative, interesting, and insightful. If you happen to have enjoyed this book, please leave a comment for me in the comment section on Amazon.

REFERENCES

Akkawi, D. (2018, August 16). *How come Zamzam's well is never depleted?* EgyptToday. https://www.egypttoday.com/Article/1/56092/How-come-Zamzam%E2%80%99s-well-is-never-depleted

Blush & Pine Creative. (2019, April 29). *Quantum jumping with the two cup method*. Blush & Pine Creative. https://blushandpinecreative.com/quantum-jumping-two-cup-method/

Chu, C. (2020, August 27). *Healing with water and energy*. Reiki, Numerology and Intuitive Energy Healing in Hong Kong | Corie Chu Healing. https://coriechu.com/blog/healing-with-water-and-energy

Fedrizzi, A., & Proietti, M. (2011, November 14). *Quantum physics: our study suggests objective reality doesn't exist*. The Conversation.

https://theconversation.com/quantum-physics-our-study-suggests-objective-reality-doesnt-exist-126805

Ismail, S. (2020, October 12). *The 7 universal laws of the universe and how to use them to create a better life.* Medium. https://medium.com/illumination/the-7-universal-laws-of-the-universe-and-how-to-use-them-to-create-a-better-lfe-a621caee77e2

Marianne. (2017, February 5). *Physics in a minute: The double slit experiment.* Plus.Maths.org. https://plus.maths.org/content/physics-minute-double-slit-experiment-0

Merriam Webster. (2020a). *Definition of QUANTUM ENTANGLEMENT.* Merriam-Webster.com. https://www.merriam-webster.com/dictionary/quantum%20entanglement

Merriam Webster. (2020b). *Merriam-Webster Dictionary | Quantum Theory.* Merriam-Webster.com. https://www.merriam-webster.com/dictionary/quantum%20theory

Mitte Team. (2019, October 14). *The curious study of water consciousness.* Mitte. https://mitte.co/2019/10/14/the-curious-study-of-water-consciousness/

Staff Writer Al Arabiya. (2018, August 16). *Hajj pilgrims consume eight mln liters of Zamzam water.* Al

Arabiya English. https://english.alarabiya.net/en/News/gulf/2018/08/16/Hajj-pilgrims-consume-8-mln-liters-of-Zamzam-water

TEDxCERN, & Barbosa, M. (2014). The weirdness of water could be the answer | Marcia Barbosa [YouTube]. In *TEDxCERN*.

The Spirit of Life. (n.d.). *Hado, the energy of life*. The Spirit of Water. https://thespiritofwater.com/pages/hado-the-energy-of-life

USGS Science for a changing world. (2019). *The water in you: Water and the human body*. Usgs.Gov. https://www.usgs.gov/special-topic/water-science-school/science/water-you-water-and-human-body

Wexler, A. (2016, April 21). *TEDxStendenUniversity | TED | Without Borders*. Www.Ted.com. https://www.ted.com/tedx/events/19105

Printed in Great Britain
by Amazon